The Gut Health Diet

Healing Recipes for Digestive Disorders and Microbiome Balance

Irma Govan

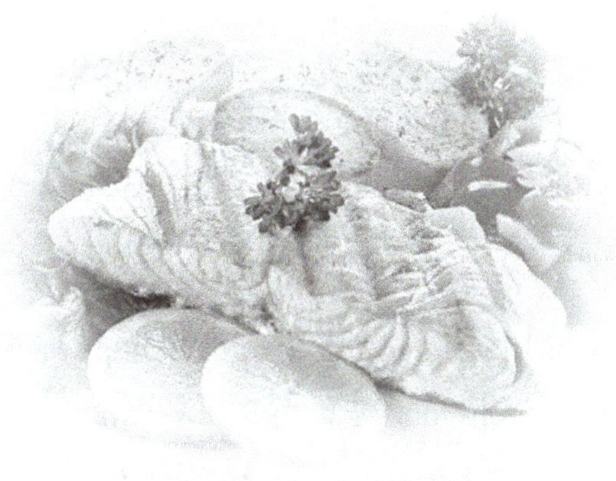

1

Copyright© Irma Govan

The author, [Irma Govan], has provided this book in an effort to provide the reader with accurate and up-to-date information. The content of this book is for information purposes only, and is not intended as medical advice or to substitute for medical advice from a physician or healthcare professional.

This book is not intended to create a physician-patient relationship, nor does it replace, modify, analyze, summarize, or otherwise alter the medical advice of a licensed healthcare professional. While reasonable efforts have been made to ensure the accuracy and completeness of the information presented, the author and publisher assume no responsibility for

Table of content

INTRODUCTION

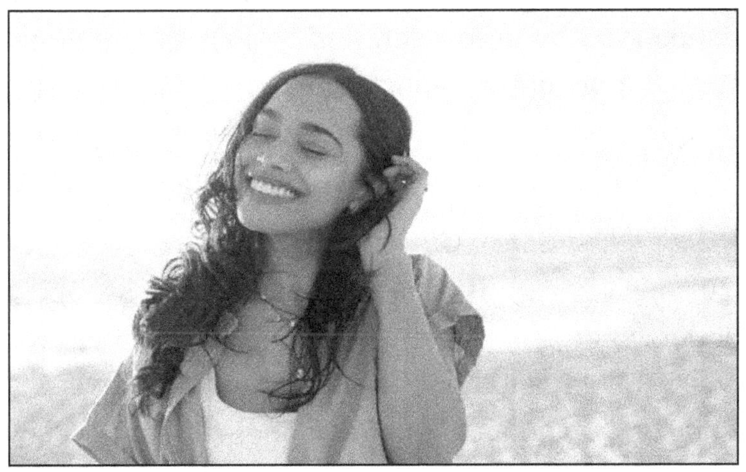

Welcome to the culinary journey that will not only tantalize your taste buds but also nurture your inner well-being. In the pages that follow, "The Gut Health Diet: Healing Recipes for Digestive Disorders and Microbiome Balance" we embark on a gastronomic adventure that celebrates the power of food as medicine.

In today's fast-paced world, digestive disorders have become all too common, often leaving us feeling uncomfortable and fatigued. But fear not, for the key to restoring your digestive health may be as close as your kitchen. This book is your compass to navigate the world of nutritious, delicious, and healing cuisine.

We believe that eating for better gut health should never mean sacrificing flavor. Here, you'll find a collection of carefully crafted recipes that not only soothe and support your digestive system but also delight your palate. From soul-warming bone broths to vibrant salads bursting with nutrients, each recipe is a step towards a healthier you.

But this journey isn't just about recipes; it's about understanding the incredible connection between what you eat and how you feel. You'll discover the science behind the ingredients, the benefits they offer, and how they can help restore balance within.

So, whether you're struggling with digestive discomfort or simply seeking to maintain a vibrant gut, "The Gut Health Diet" is your trusted companion.

Together, let's explore the flavors, textures, and wholesome goodness that not only heal but also nourish, making every meal a step towards a healthier, happier you. Let's begin the transformative voyage to better gut health, one delectable bite at a time.

Recipe 1: Soothing Bone Broth

Ingredients:

- 2 lbs grass-fed beef bones
- 1 onion, peeled and halved
- 2 carrots, chopped
- 2 celery stalks, chopped
- 3 cloves garlic, smashed
- 1-inch piece of ginger, sliced
- 1 tablespoon apple cider vinegar
- Salt and pepper to taste
- Fresh herbs (thyme, rosemary) for garnish (optional)

Instructions:

1. Preheat your oven to 400°F (200°C).
2. Place beef bones on a baking sheet and roast for 20 minutes.
3. Transfer bones to a large pot, add onion, carrots, celery, garlic, and ginger.
4. Cover with water, add apple cider vinegar, and bring to a gentle simmer.

5. Skim off all foams that have risen to the top. Simmer for 12-24 hours.

6. Strain the broth, and season with salt and pepper.

7. If preferred, serve hot with fresh herbs as a garnish.

Recipe 2: Healing Ginger Tea

Ingredients:

- 1-inch piece of ginger, sliced

- 2 cups water

- 1 teaspoon honey (optional)

- Squeeze of lemon juice (optional)

Instructions:

1. Add slices of ginger to a boiling water

2. Let it simmer for 10-15 minutes.

3. Strain into a cup.

4. Add honey and lemon juice to taste.

Recipe 3: Creamy Banana Oatmeal

Ingredients:

- 1 cup rolled oats

- 2 cups water or milk (dairy-free alternatives work)

- 2 ripe bananas, mashed

- 1 tablespoon chia seeds

- Cinnamon to taste

- Toppings: Sliced bananas, chopped nuts

Instructions:

1. Combine oats and water/milk in a pot, cook until creamy.

2. Stir in mashed bananas and chia seeds.

3. Add cinnamon to taste.

4. Serve hot, topped with sliced bananas and nuts.

Recipe 4: Roasted Carrot and Ginger Soup

Ingredients:

- 4 large carrots, peeled and chopped

- 1 onion, chopped

- 2 cloves garlic, minced

- peel and mince an inch piece of ginger

- 4 cups vegetable broth

- 2 tablespoons olive oil

- Salt and pepper to taste

- Fresh cilantro for garnish (optional)

Instructions:

1. Preheat oven to 425°F (220°C).

2. Toss carrots with olive oil, and roast for 25-30 minutes.

3. In a pot, sauté onion, garlic, and ginger until fragrant.

4. Add roasted carrots and vegetable broth. Simmer for 15 minutes.

5. Blend to a smoother texture, season with salt and pepper.

6. Serve hot, garnished with fresh cilantro if desired.

Recipe 5: Quinoa and Grilled Chicken Bowl

Ingredients:

- 1 cup quinoa, rinsed

- 2 cups water or broth

- 2 boneless, skinless chicken breasts

- 1 tablespoon olive oil

- 1 teaspoon paprika

- Salt and pepper to taste

- Mixed greens

- Sliced cucumber, tomatoes, and bell peppers

- Lemon-tahini dressing

Instructions:

1. Cook quinoa in water/broth according to package instructions.

2. Rub chicken with olive oil, paprika, salt, and pepper.

3. Grill chicken until cooked through, slice.

4. Assemble bowls with quinoa, mixed greens, sliced chicken, and veggies.

5. Drizzle with lemon-tahini dressing.

Recipe 6: Baked Salmon with Turmeric

Ingredients:

- 2 salmon fillets

- 1 teaspoon turmeric

- 1 teaspoon paprika

- 1 tablespoon olive oil

- Salt and pepper to taste

- Lemon wedges

- Fresh parsley for garnish (optional)

Instructions:

1. Preheat oven to 375°F (190°C).

2. Mix turmeric, paprika, olive oil, salt, and pepper in a bowl.

3. Coat salmon fillets with the spice mixture.

4. Place fillets on a baking sheet and bake for 15-20 minutes.

5. Garnish with fresh parsley and serve with lemon segments.

Recipe 7: Gut-Healing Smoothie

Ingredients:

- 1 cup unsweetened kefir or yogurt (dairy-free alternatives work)

- 1 cup frozen mixed berries

- 1 small banana

- 1 tablespoon chia seeds

- 1 tablespoon honey (optional)

- ½ teaspoon grated ginger

Instructions:

1. Blend kefir/yogurt, mixed berries, banana, chia seeds, honey, and ginger until smooth.

2. Adjust thickness by adding water if needed.

3. Pour into a glass and enjoy it as a nutritious smoothie.

Recipe 8: Easy Mashed Sweet Potatoes

Ingredients:

- 2 large sweet potatoes, peeled and cubed

- 2 tablespoons coconut oil

- ¼ cup unsweetened almond milk

- 1 teaspoon cinnamon

- Salt to taste

- Chopped green onions for garnish (optional)

Instructions:

1. Boil or steam sweet potato cubes until tender, drain.

2. Mash with coconut oil, almond milk, cinnamon, and salt.

3. Adjust consistency to your liking with more almond milk.

4. Serve hot, garnished with chopped green onions.

Recipe 9: Sautéed Spinach with Garlic

Ingredients:

- 1 bunch of washed and drained fresh spinach

- 2 cloves garlic, minced

- 1 tablespoon olive oil

- Salt and pepper to taste

- Lemon zest (optional)

Instructions:

1. In a skillet, heat the olive oil and sauté the minced garlic until fragrant.

2. Add spinach, and cook until wilted.

3. Sprinkle some salt, pepper, and lemon zest if using.

4. Serve as a nutritious side dish.

Recipe 10: Berry Chia Seed Pudding

Ingredients:

- ½ cup mixed berries (fresh or frozen)

- 2 tablespoons chia seeds

- 1 cup unsweetened coconut milk

- ½ teaspoon vanilla extract

- 1 tablespoon honey (optional)

- Sliced almonds for topping

Instructions:

1. Blend mixed berries until smooth.

2. Mix berry puree, chia seeds, coconut milk, vanilla, and honey (if using).

3. To thicken, place in the refrigerator for at least 2 hours or overnight.

4. Serve in small bowls, topped with sliced almonds.

Recipe 11: Zucchini Noodles with Pesto

Ingredients:

- 2 medium zucchinis, spiralized

- ½ cup fresh basil leaves

- ¼ cup pine nuts

- 2 cloves garlic

- ¼ cup grated Parmesan cheese (optional)

- ¼ cup olive oil

- Salt and pepper to taste

Instructions:

1. Blend basil, pine nuts, garlic, and Parmesan (if using) in a food processor.

2. Slowly add olive oil to form a pesto sauce. Season with salt and pepper.

3. Toss zucchini noodles with pesto and serve.

Recipe 12: Healing Turmeric Latte

Ingredients:

- 1 cup almond milk (or milk of choice)

- ½ teaspoon turmeric

- ½ teaspoon cinnamon

- Pinch of black pepper (increases turmeric absorption)

- 1 teaspoon honey or maple syrup (optional)

Instructions:

1. Warm almond milk in a small pot.

2. Whisk in turmeric, cinnamon, and black pepper.

3. Sweeten with honey or maple syrup if desired.

4. Pour into a mug and enjoy.

Recipe 13: Roasted Brussels Sprouts

Ingredients:

- 1 lb Brussels sprouts, trimmed and halved

- 2 tablespoons olive oil

- 1 teaspoon garlic powder

- Salt and pepper to taste

Instructions:

1. Preheat oven to 400°F (200°C).

2. Toss Brussels sprouts with olive oil and garlic seasoning.

3. Roast for 20-25 minutes, until crispy and translucent.

4. Season with salt and pepper before serving.

Recipe 14: Gut-Healing Miso Soup

Ingredients:

- 4 cups vegetable broth

- 2 tablespoons miso paste

- 1 cup sliced mushrooms

- 1 cup diced tofu

- 2 green onions, sliced

- 1 teaspoon grated ginger

Instructions:

1. Heat vegetable broth in a pot until hot but not boiling.

2. In a small bowl, whisk miso paste with a bit of hot broth until smooth.

3. Add miso mixture, mushrooms, and tofu to the pot. Simmer gently.

4. Stir in green onions and grated ginger.

5. Serve hot.

Recipe 15: Creamy Avocado Salad Dressing

Ingredients:

- 1 ripe avocado, peeled and pitted

- ¼ cup plain Greek yogurt

- 2 tablespoons lime juice

- 2 tablespoons olive oil

- 1 clove garlic, minced

- Salt and pepper to taste

- Water to adjust consistency

  Instructions:

1. Blend avocado, Greek yogurt, lime juice, olive oil, and garlic.

2. Add water to reach the desired consistency.

3. Season with salt and pepper.

4. Drizzle over salads or use as a dip.

Recipe 16: Easy Baked Apples

Ingredients:

- 4 apples, cored and halved

- 2 tablespoons melted coconut oil

- 2 tablespoons honey

- ½ teaspoon cinnamon

- ¼ cup chopped walnuts

Instructions:

1. Preheat oven to 350°F (175°C).

2. Place apple halves in a baking dish.

3. Mix melted coconut oil, honey, and cinnamon.

4. Drizzle mixture over apples. Sprinkle with chopped walnuts.

5. Bake for 20-25 minutes until the apples become soft.

Recipe 17: Gingered Carrot and Apple Salad

Ingredients:

- 2 cups grated carrots

- 1 apple, thinly sliced

- 2 tablespoons chopped fresh cilantro

- 1 tablespoon grated ginger

- 2 tablespoons olive oil

- 1 tablespoon apple cider vinegar

- Salt and pepper to taste

Instructions:

1. Combine grated carrots, apple slices, and cilantro in a bowl.

2. In a separate bowl, whisk grated ginger, olive oil, and apple cider vinegar.

3. Toss dressing with the carrot-apple mixture.

4. Season with salt and pepper.

Recipe 18: Lemon Garlic Roasted Chicken

Ingredients:

- 4 bone-in, skin-on chicken thighs

- 2 tablespoons olive oil

- Juice and zest of 1 lemon

- 3 cloves garlic, minced

- 1 teaspoon dried thyme

- Salt and pepper to taste

Instructions:

1. Preheat oven to 425°F (220°C).

2. Mix olive oil, lemon juice, lemon zest, minced garlic, and thyme.

3. Rub mixture over chicken thighs. Season with salt and pepper.

4. Roast in the oven for 25-30 minutes until heated through.

Recipe 19: Roasted Beet and Goat Cheese Salad

Ingredients:

- 4 medium beets, peeled and cubed

- 2 cups mixed salad greens

- ½ cup crumbled goat cheese

- ¼ cup chopped walnuts

- Balsamic vinaigrette

Instructions:

1. Preheat oven to 375°F (190°C).

2. Toss beet cubes with olive oil and roast for 25-30 minutes.

3. Arrange salad greens on plates, and and top with roasted beets, goat cheese, and walnuts.

4. Drizzle with balsamic vinaigrette.

Recipe 20: Gut-Healing Kombucha Mocktail

Ingredients:

- 1 cup kombucha (flavor of your choice)

- ½ cup sparkling water

- Squeeze of lemon or lime juice

- Fresh mint leaves for garnish

Instructions:

1. Fill a glass with ice.

2. Pour kombucha and sparkling water over the ice.

3. Squeeze in some lemon or lime juice.

4. Garnish with fresh mint leaves after gently stirring.

Recipe 21: Cumin-Spiced Cauliflower Rice

Ingredients:

- 1 head cauliflower, grated into rice-like texture

- 2 tablespoons olive oil

- 1 teaspoon ground cumin

- ½ teaspoon ground turmeric

- Salt and pepper to taste

- Fresh cilantro for garnish

Instructions:

1. Heat olive oil in a pan, add cauliflower rice.

2. Sauté for 5-7 minutes until tender.

3. Stir in ground cumin, ground turmeric, salt,
    and pepper.

4. Garnish with fresh cilantro before serving.

Recipe 22: Herbed Baked Cod

Ingredients:

- 4 cod fillets

- 2 tablespoons melted butter or ghee

- 2 tablespoons chopped fresh herbs (such as
  parsley, dill, thyme)

- Juice of 1 lemon

- Salt and pepper to taste

Instructions:

1. Preheat oven to 400°F (200°C).

2. Place cod fillets on a baking sheet.

3. Mix melted butter/ghee, chopped herbs, and
    lemon juice.

4. Drizzle mixture over cod. Season with salt
    and pepper.

5. Cook for 12-15 minutes, or until the fish
    flakes easily.

Recipe 23: Blueberry Chia Jam

Ingredients:

- 2 cups fresh or frozen blueberries
- 2 tablespoons chia seeds
- 1-2 tablespoons honey or maple syrup
- ½ teaspoon vanilla extract

Instructions:

1. In a saucepan, heat blueberries until they start to release juices.
2. Mash blueberries with a fork or potato masher.
3. Stir in chia seeds, honey/maple syrup, and vanilla extract.
4. Cook for a few minutes longer, or until the jam starts to thick.
5. Let cool and then transfer to a jar.

Recipe 24: Coconut Yogurt Parfait

Ingredients:

- 1 cup coconut yogurt
- ½ cup granola
- ½ cup mixed berries
- 2 tablespoons shredded coconut
- Drizzle of honey (optional)

Instructions:

1. Layer coconut yogurt, granola, and mixed berries in a glass.

2. Repeat the layers.
3. Top with shredded coconut and a drizzle of honey if desired.

Recipe 25: Mediterranean Chickpea Salad

Ingredients:
- 2 cups cooked chickpeas
- 1 cucumber, diced
- 1 cup cherry tomatocs, halved
- ½ red onion, finely chopped
- ½ cup chopped fresh parsley
- ¼ cup crumbled feta cheese
- 3 tablespoons olive oil
- Juice of 1 lemon
- 1 teaspoon dried oregano
- Salt and pepper to taste

Instructions:
1. Combine chickpeas, cucumber, cherry tomatoes, red onion, parsley, and feta cheese.
2. In a separate bowl, whisk olive oil, lemon juice, dried oregano, salt, and pepper.
3. Toss dressing with the chickpea mixture.
4. Serve as a refreshing salad.

Recipe 26: Spinach and Mushroom Omelette

Ingredients:

- 3 eggs
- ½ cup sliced mushrooms
- 1 cup fresh spinach leaves
- 2 tablespoons grated cheese (optional)
- Salt and pepper to taste
- 1 teaspoon olive oil or butter

Instructions:

1. Heat olive oil/butter in a pan.
2. Sauté mushrooms until browned.
3. Add spinach and cook until wilted.
4. Beat eggs, season with salt and pepper.
5. Pour eggs over veggies, and cook until set.
6. Sprinkle cheese on one half, afterwards fold over the other.
7. Cook until cheese melts.

Recipe 27: Roasted Garlic Hummus

Ingredients:

- 1 can (15 oz) cleaned and drained chickpeas
- 1 head garlic
- ¼ cup tahini
- 2 tablespoons olive oil
- Juice of 1 lemon

- Salt and pepper to taste
- Paprika and olive oil for garnish

Instructions:

1. Preheat oven to 400°F (200°C).
2. Cut the top off the garlic head, drizzle with olive oil, and wrap in foil.
3. Toast the garlic cloves for 30-35 minutes, or until they become soft.
4. Squeeze and put roasted garlic cloves in a food processor.
5. Add chickpeas, tahini, olive oil, lemon juice, salt, and pepper.
6. Blend until smooth. Adjust seasoning.
7. Serve with a sprinkle of paprika and olive oil drizzle.

Recipe 28: Baked Quinoa-Stuffed Bell Peppers

Ingredients:

- halve four bell peppers and remove seeds
- 1 cup cooked quinoa
- 1 cup cooked black beans
- 1 cup diced tomatoes
- 1 cup diced zucchini
- 1 teaspoon cumin
- 1 teaspoon chili powder
- Salt and pepper to taste

- ½ cup shredded cheddar cheese (optional)

Instructions:

1. Preheat oven to 375°F (190°C).
2. Mix cooked quinoa, black beans, diced tomatoes, diced zucchini, cumin, chili powder, salt, and pepper.
3. Fill bell pepper halves with the quinoa mixture.
4. Place peppers in a baking dish. Cover with foil.
5. Bake for 25-30 minutes, or until peppers look tender or translucent.
6. If using cheese, sprinkle on top and bake uncovered for an additional 5 minutes.

Recipe 29: Banana Walnut Muffins

Ingredients:

- 1 ½ cups whole wheat flour
- 1 teaspoon baking soda
- ¼ teaspoon salt
- 3 ripe bananas, mashed
- ¼ cup honey or maple syrup
- 1 egg
- 1 teaspoon vanilla extract
- ½ cup chopped walnuts

Instructions:

1. Preheat oven to 350°F (175°C). Prepare a muffin pan using paper liners.
2. In a mixing bowl, combine the flour, baking soda, and salt.
3. In another bowl, mix mashed bananas, honey/maple syrup, egg, and vanilla.
4. Combine wet and dry ingredients. Stir in chopped walnuts.
5. Divide batter among muffin cups.
6. Bake for 18-20 minutes, or until the toothpick inserted into the center comes out clean.

Recipe 30: Ginger-turmeric granola Bars

Ingredients:

- 1 ½ cups rolled oats
- ½ cup of chopped nuts (walnuts, almonds, etc.)
- ¼ cup dried fruits (raisins, apricots, etc.)
- 2 tablespoons chia seeds
- 1 teaspoon ground ginger
- ½ teaspoon ground turmeric
- ¼ cup honey or maple syrup
- ¼ cup of nut butter (almond, peanut, etc.)
- 1 teaspoon vanilla extract

Instructions:

1. Preheat oven to 350°F (175°C). Using sheets of parchment paper, line a baking pan.
2. In a bowl, mix oats, chopped nuts, dried fruits, chia seeds, ginger, and turmeric.
3. In a saucepan, warm honey/maple syrup, nut butter, and vanilla.
4. Combine wet and dry ingredients. Press into the baking pan.
5. Bake for 15-20 minutes, or until the edges tend to be golden brown.
6. Let cool before cutting into bars.

Recipe 31: Creamy Cauliflower Soup

Ingredients:

- 1 head cauliflower, chopped
- 1 onion, chopped
- 2 cloves garlic, minced
- 4 cups vegetable broth
- ½ cup coconut milk
- 2 tablespoons olive oil
- Salt and pepper to taste
- Fresh parsley for garnish

Instructions:

1. Sauté onion and garlic in olive oil in a pot until translucent and aromatic

2. Add chopped cauliflower and vegetable broth. Simmer until cauliflower is tender.
3. Blend the mixture until smooth. Return to the pot.
4. Season with salt and pepper and mix in the coconut milk.
5. Heat the soup gently. Serve hot, garnished with fresh parsley.

Conclusion

As we close the pages of "The Gut Health Diet: Healing Recipes for Digestive Disorders and Microbiome Balance," we hope you've embarked on a transformative culinary journey—one that has not only expanded your palate but also enhanced your well-being. Through these pages, we've explored the profound connection between the foods wc consume and the vitality we experience.

In this concluding chapter, we want to remind you that the recipes within this book are not just a collection of ingredients and instructions. They are tools for healing and nourishment, for bringing harmony to your digestive system, and for rekindling your love for wholesome, flavorful food.

Your gut health is a lifelong journey, and this book is but a stepping stone. As you continue to experiment with these recipes and explore the world of digestive wellness, remember the wisdom of balance. Cherish the knowledge that every bite holds the potential to heal and nurture.

Digestive disorders may challenge us, but they also empower us to make mindful choices about what we eat and how we care for ourselves. This book is your companion in that journey, offering guidance, inspiration, and the assurance that you can take control of your health through the simple act of cooking.

We encourage you to keep experimenting, to try new ingredients, and to listen to your body. Discover what works best for you, and relish the benefits of a harmonious gut. Share these recipes with loved ones, spread the joy of nourishment, and let your kitchen become a sanctuary for wellness.

Above all, remember that this book is not an endpoint but a beginning—a foundation upon which you can build a lifetime of vibrant health. We are honored to have been part of your journey, and we wish you a future filled with delicious, healing meals and boundless well-being.

Thank you for joining us on this adventure. May your path to gut health be rich with flavor, vitality, and joy. Here's to a future filled with good food and great health. Bon appétit!